This Journal Belongs To:

_____

Progress Tracker

Chest

Arm

Waist

Hips

Thigh

STARTING MEASUREMENTS:

WEIGHT:

LEFT ARM:

RIGHT ARM:

CHEST:

WAIST:

HIPS:

LEFT THIGH:

RIGHT THIGH:

My Journey

PERSONAL GOALS:

Meal Planner

MONDAY	NOTES

TUESDAY	NOTES

WEDNESDAY	NOTES

THURSDAY	NOTES

FRIDAY	NOTES

Meal Planner

SATURDAY

NOTES

SUNDAY

NOTES

MY PROGRESS:

My Workout Routine

DATE:

ACTIVITY:

TIME:

DISTANCE:

SETS:

REPS:

WEIGHT USED:

CALORIES BURNED:

WATER INTAKE:

My Routine

Progress Tracker

CURRENT:

PREVIOUS:

CHANGE:

NOTES

One day at a time...

Meal Planner

DATE:

BREAKFAST:

_____

_____

_____

LUNCH:

_____

_____

_____

DINNER:

_____

_____

_____

SNACKS:

_____

_____

_____

_____

Progress Tracker

DATE:

	MEASUREMENT:	LOSS/GAIN:
WEIGHT:		
LEFT ARM:		
RIGHT ARM:		
CHEST:		
WAIST:		
HIPS:		
LEFT THIGH:		
RIGHT THIGH:		

Weekly Goals

Meal Planner

	BREAKFAST	LUNCH	DINNER
MON			
TUES			
WED			
THU			
FRI			
SAT			
SUN			

Progress Tracker

Chest

Arm

Waist

Hips

Thigh

STARTING MEASUREMENTS:

WEIGHT:

LEFT ARM:

RIGHT ARM:

CHEST:

WAIST:

HIPS:

LEFT THIGH:

RIGHT THIGH:

My Journey

PERSONAL GOALS:

Meal Planner

MONDAY

NOTES

TUESDAY

NOTES

WEDNESDAY

NOTES

THURSDAY

NOTES

FRIDAY

NOTES

Meal Planner

SATURDAY

NOTES

SUNDAY

NOTES

MY PROGRESS:

My Workout Routine

DATE:

ACTIVITY:

TIME:

DISTANCE:

SETS:

REPS:

WEIGHT USED:

CALORIES BURNED:

WATER INTAKE:

My Routine

Progress Tracker

CURRENT:

PREVIOUS:

CHANGE:

NOTES

One day at a time…

Meal Planner

DATE:

BREAKFAST:

_____

_____

LUNCH:

_____

_____

DINNER:

_____

_____

SNACKS:

_____

_____

_____

_____

Progress Tracker

DATE:

	MEASUREMENT:	LOSS/GAIN:
WEIGHT:		
LEFT ARM:		
RIGHT ARM:		
CHEST:		
WAIST:		
HIPS:		
LEFT THIGH:		
RIGHT THIGH:		

Weekly Goals

Meal Planner

	BREAKFAST	LUNCH	DINNER
MON			
TUES			
WED			
THU			
FRI			
SAT			
SUN			

Progress Tracker

Chest

Arm

Waist

Hips

Thigh

STARTING MEASUREMENTS:

WEIGHT:
LEFT ARM:
RIGHT ARM:
CHEST:
WAIST:
HIPS:
LEFT THIGH:
RIGHT THIGH:

My Journey

PERSONAL GOALS:

Meal Planner

MONDAY

NOTES

TUESDAY

NOTES

WEDNESDAY

NOTES

THURSDAY

NOTES

FRIDAY

NOTES

Meal Planner

SATURDAY

NOTES

SUNDAY

NOTES

MY PROGRESS:

My Workout Routine

DATE:

ACTIVITY:

TIME:

DISTANCE:

SETS:

REPS:

WEIGHT USED:

CALORIES BURNED:

WATER INTAKE:

My Routine

Progress Tracker

CURRENT:

PREVIOUS:

CHANGE:

NOTES

One day at a time…

Meal Planner

DATE:

BREAKFAST:

LUNCH:

DINNER:

SNACKS:

Progress Tracker

DATE:

	MEASUREMENT:	LOSS/GAIN:
WEIGHT:		
LEFT ARM:		
RIGHT ARM:		
CHEST:		
WAIST:		
HIPS:		
LEFT THIGH:		
RIGHT THIGH:		

Weekly Goals

Meal Planner

	BREAKFAST	LUNCH	DINNER
MON			
TUES			
WED			
THU			
FRI			
SAT			
SUN			

Progress Tracker

Chest

Arm

Waist

Hips

Thigh

STARTING MEASUREMENTS:

WEIGHT:

LEFT ARM:

RIGHT ARM:

CHEST:

WAIST:

HIPS:

LEFT THIGH:

RIGHT THIGH:

My Journey

PERSONAL GOALS:

Meal Planner

MONDAY

NOTES

TUESDAY

NOTES

WEDNESDAY

NOTES

THURSDAY

NOTES

FRIDAY

NOTES

Meal Planner

SATURDAY

NOTES

SUNDAY

NOTES

MY PROGRESS:

My Workout Routine

DATE:

ACTIVITY:

TIME:

DISTANCE:

SETS:

REPS:

WEIGHT USED:

CALORIES BURNED:

WATER INTAKE:

My Routine

Progress Tracker

CURRENT:

PREVIOUS:

CHANGE:

NOTES

One day at a time…

Meal Planner

DATE:

BREAKFAST:

LUNCH:

DINNER:

SNACKS:

Progress Tracker

DATE:

	MEASUREMENT:	LOSS/GAIN:
WEIGHT:		
LEFT ARM:		
RIGHT ARM:		
CHEST:		
WAIST:		
HIPS:		
LEFT THIGH:		
RIGHT THIGH:		

Weekly Goals

Meal Planner

	BREAKFAST	LUNCH	DINNER
MON			
TUES			
WED			
THU			
FRI			
SAT			
SUN			

Progress Tracker

Chest

Arm

Waist

Hips

Thigh

WEIGHT:

LEFT ARM:

RIGHT ARM:

CHEST:

WAIST:

HIPS:

LEFT THIGH:

RIGHT THIGH:

My Journey

PERSONAL GOALS:

Meal Planner

MONDAY

NOTES

TUESDAY

NOTES

WEDNESDAY

NOTES

THURSDAY

NOTES

FRIDAY

NOTES

Meal Planner

SATURDAY

NOTES

SUNDAY

NOTES

MY PROGRESS:

My Workout Routine

DATE:

ACTIVITY:

TIME:

DISTANCE:

SETS:

REPS:

WEIGHT USED:

CALORIES BURNED:

WATER INTAKE:

My Routine

Progress Tracker

CURRENT:

PREVIOUS:

CHANGE:

NOTES

One day at a time…

Meal Planner

DATE:

BREAKFAST:

LUNCH:

DINNER:

SNACKS:

Progress Tracker

DATE:

	MEASUREMENT:	LOSS/GAIN:
WEIGHT:		
LEFT ARM:		
RIGHT ARM:		
CHEST:		
WAIST:		
HIPS:		
LEFT THIGH:		
RIGHT THIGH:		

Weekly Goals

Meal Planner

	BREAKFAST	LUNCH	DINNER
MON			
TUES			
WED			
THU			
FRI			
SAT			
SUN			

Progress Tracker

Chest

Arm

Waist

Hips

Thigh

WEIGHT:
LEFT ARM:
RIGHT ARM:
CHEST:
WAIST:
HIPS:
LEFT THIGH:
RIGHT THIGH:

My Journey

PERSONAL GOALS:

Meal Planner

MONDAY

NOTES

TUESDAY

NOTES

WEDNESDAY

NOTES

THURSDAY

NOTES

FRIDAY

NOTES

Meal Planner

SATURDAY

NOTES

SUNDAY

NOTES

MY PROGRESS:

My Workout Routine

DATE:

ACTIVITY:

TIME:

DISTANCE:

SETS:

REPS:

WEIGHT USED:

CALORIES BURNED:

WATER INTAKE:

My Routine

Progress Tracker

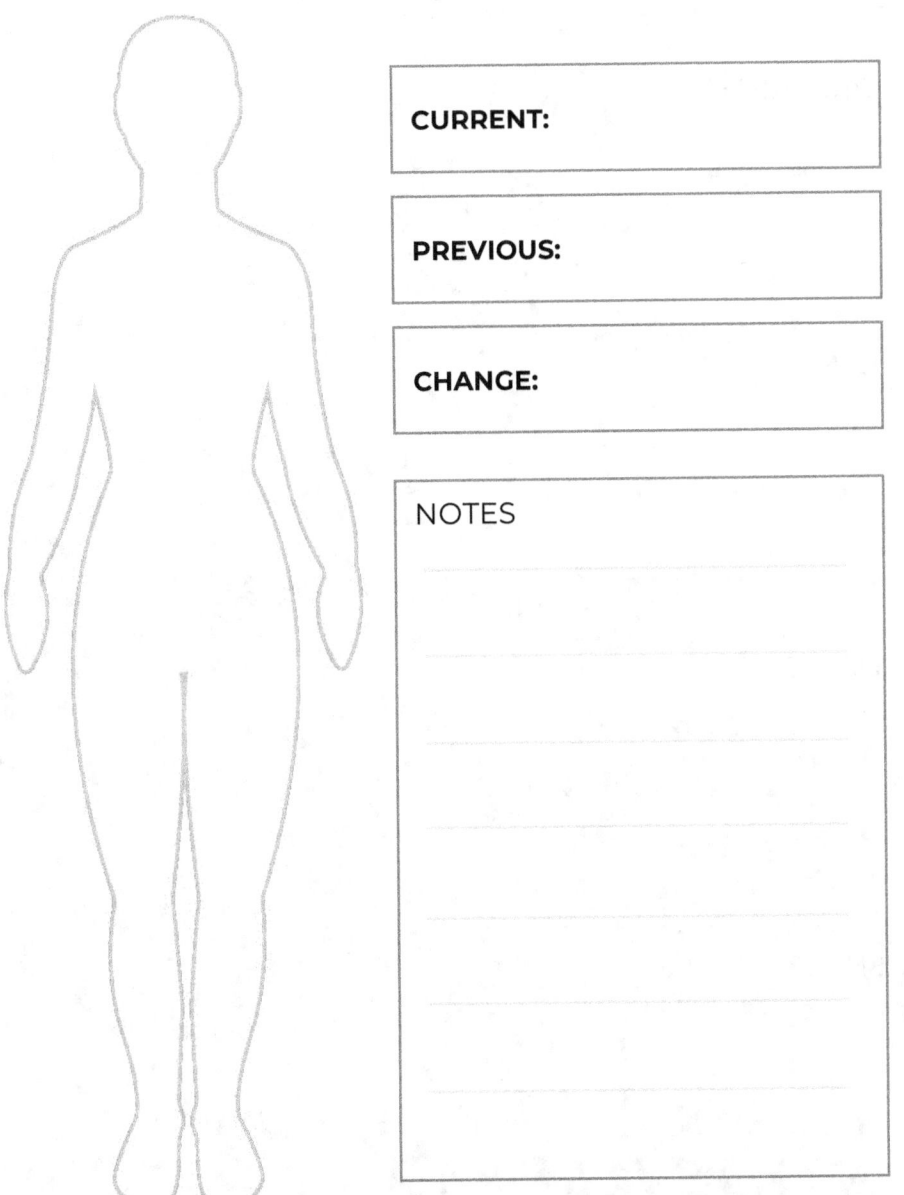

CURRENT:

PREVIOUS:

CHANGE:

NOTES

One day at a time…

Meal Planner

DATE:

BREAKFAST:

LUNCH:

DINNER:

SNACKS:

Progress Tracker

DATE:

	MEASUREMENT:	LOSS/GAIN:
WEIGHT:		
LEFT ARM:		
RIGHT ARM:		
CHEST:		
WAIST:		
HIPS:		
LEFT THIGH:		
RIGHT THIGH:		

Weekly Goals

Meal Planner

	BREAKFAST	LUNCH	DINNER
MON			
TUES			
WED			
THU			
FRI			
SAT			
SUN			

Progress Tracker

Chest

Arm

Waist

Hips

Thigh

STARTING MEASUREMENTS:

WEIGHT:

LEFT ARM:

RIGHT ARM:

CHEST:

WAIST:

HIPS:

LEFT THIGH:

RIGHT THIGH:

My Journey

PERSONAL GOALS:

Meal Planner

MONDAY

NOTES

TUESDAY

NOTES

WEDNESDAY

NOTES

THURSDAY

NOTES

FRIDAY

NOTES

Meal Planner

SATURDAY

NOTES

SUNDAY

NOTES

MY PROGRESS:

My Workout Routine

DATE:

ACTIVITY:

TIME:

DISTANCE:

SETS:

REPS:

WEIGHT USED:

CALORIES BURNED:

WATER INTAKE:

My Routine

Progress Tracker

CURRENT:

PREVIOUS:

CHANGE:

NOTES

One day at a time...

Meal Planner

DATE:

BREAKFAST:

_____

_____

_____

LUNCH:

_____

_____

_____

DINNER:

_____

_____

_____

SNACKS:

_____

_____

_____

_____

Progress Tracker

DATE:

	MEASUREMENT:	LOSS/GAIN:
WEIGHT:		
LEFT ARM:		
RIGHT ARM:		
CHEST:		
WAIST:		
HIPS:		
LEFT THIGH:		
RIGHT THIGH:		

Weekly Goals

Meal Planner

	BREAKFAST	LUNCH	DINNER
MON			
TUES			
WED			
THU			
FRI			
SAT			
SUN			

Progress Tracker

Chest

Arm

Waist

Hips

Thigh

WEIGHT:

LEFT ARM:

RIGHT ARM:

CHEST:

WAIST:

HIPS:

LEFT THIGH:

RIGHT THIGH:

My Journey

PERSONAL GOALS:

Meal Planner

MONDAY

NOTES

TUESDAY

NOTES

WEDNESDAY

NOTES

THURSDAY

NOTES

FRIDAY

NOTES

Meal Planner

SATURDAY

NOTES

SUNDAY

NOTES

MY PROGRESS:

My Workout Routine

DATE:

ACTIVITY:

TIME:

DISTANCE:

SETS:

REPS:

WEIGHT USED:

CALORIES BURNED:

WATER INTAKE:

My Routine

Progress Tracker

CURRENT:

PREVIOUS:

CHANGE:

NOTES

One day at a time...

Meal Planner

DATE:

BREAKFAST:

LUNCH:

DINNER:

SNACKS:

Progress Tracker

DATE:

	MEASUREMENT:	LOSS/GAIN:
WEIGHT:		
LEFT ARM:		
RIGHT ARM:		
CHEST:		
WAIST:		
HIPS:		
LEFT THIGH:		
RIGHT THIGH:		

Weekly Goals

Meal Planner

	BREAKFAST	LUNCH	DINNER
MON			
TUES			
WED			
THU			
FRI			
SAT			
SUN			

Progress Tracker

Chest

Arm

Waist

Hips

Thigh

STARTING MEASUREMENTS:

| WEIGHT: |
| LEFT ARM: |
| RIGHT ARM: |
| CHEST: |
| WAIST: |
| HIPS: |
| LEFT THIGH: |
| RIGHT THIGH: |

My Journey

PERSONAL GOALS:

Meal Planner

MONDAY

NOTES

TUESDAY

NOTES

WEDNESDAY

NOTES

THURSDAY

NOTES

FRIDAY

NOTES

Meal Planner

SATURDAY

NOTES

SUNDAY

NOTES

MY PROGRESS:

My Workout Routine

DATE:

ACTIVITY:

TIME:

DISTANCE:

SETS:

REPS:

WEIGHT USED:

CALORIES BURNED:

WATER INTAKE:

My Routine

Progress Tracker

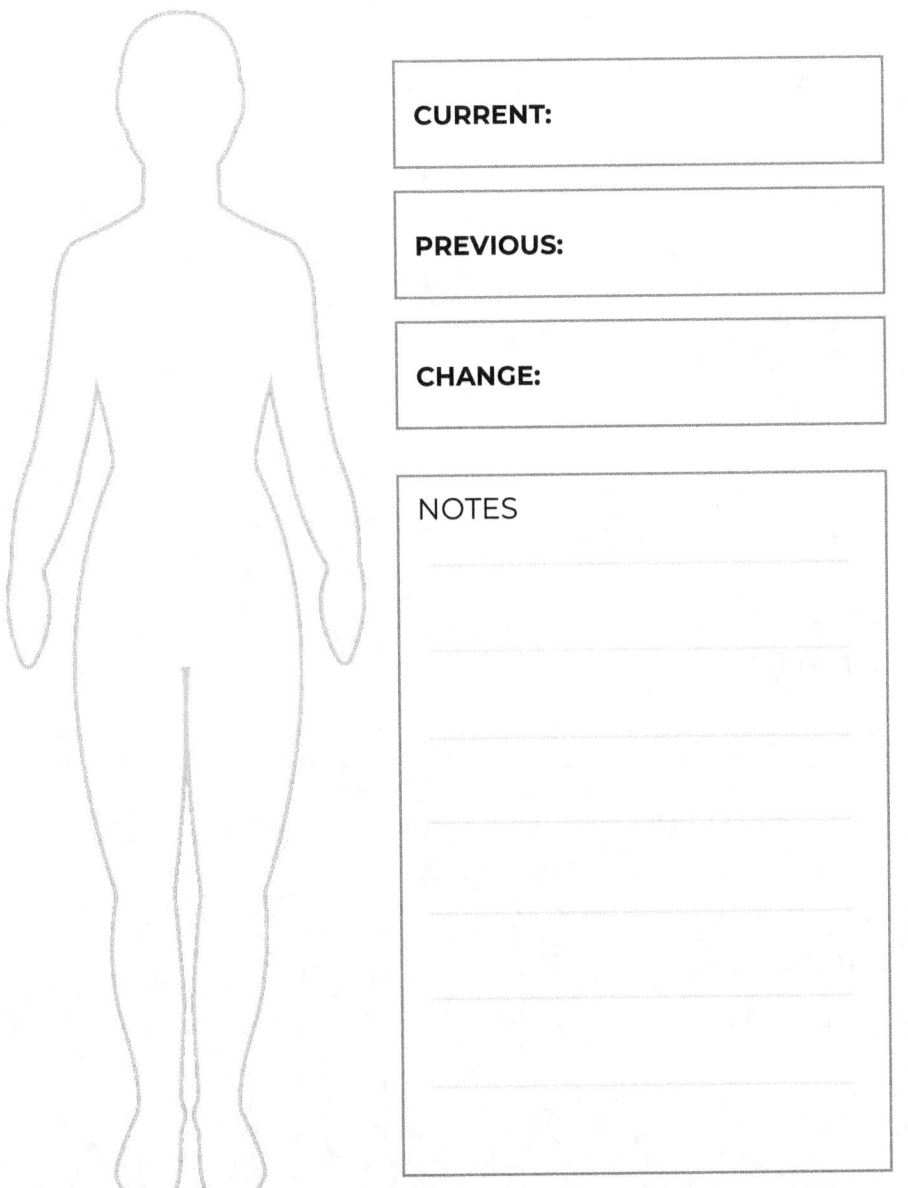

CURRENT:

PREVIOUS:

CHANGE:

NOTES

One day at a time…

Meal Planner

DATE:

BREAKFAST:

LUNCH:

DINNER:

SNACKS:

Progress Tracker

DATE:

	MEASUREMENT:	LOSS/GAIN:
WEIGHT:		
LEFT ARM:		
RIGHT ARM:		
CHEST:		
WAIST:		
HIPS:		
LEFT THIGH:		
RIGHT THIGH:		

Weekly Goals

Meal Planner

	BREAKFAST	LUNCH	DINNER
MON			
TUES			
WED			
THU			
FRI			
SAT			
SUN			

Progress Tracker

Chest

Arm

Waist

Hips

Thigh

STARTING MEASUREMENTS:

| WEIGHT: |
| LEFT ARM: |
| RIGHT ARM: |
| CHEST: |
| WAIST: |
| HIPS: |
| LEFT THIGH: |
| RIGHT THIGH: |

My Journey

PERSONAL GOALS:

Meal Planner

MONDAY

NOTES

TUESDAY

NOTES

WEDNESDAY

NOTES

THURSDAY

NOTES

FRIDAY

NOTES

Meal Planner

SATURDAY

NOTES

SUNDAY

NOTES

MY PROGRESS:

My Workout Routine

DATE:

ACTIVITY:

TIME:

DISTANCE:

SETS:

REPS:

WEIGHT USED:

CALORIES BURNED:

WATER INTAKE:

My Routine

Progress Tracker

CURRENT:

PREVIOUS:

CHANGE:

NOTES

One day at a time...

Meal Planner

DATE:

BREAKFAST:

LUNCH:

DINNER:

SNACKS:

Progress Tracker

DATE:

	MEASUREMENT:	LOSS/GAIN:
WEIGHT:		
LEFT ARM:		
RIGHT ARM:		
CHEST:		
WAIST:		
HIPS:		
LEFT THIGH:		
RIGHT THIGH:		

Weekly Goals

Meal Planner

	BREAKFAST	LUNCH	DINNER
MON			
TUES			
WED			
THU			
FRI			
SAT			
SUN			

www.ingramcontent.com/pod-product-compliance
Lightning Source LLC
Chambersburg PA
CBHW072056280526
45788CB00006B/2305